Memory, Learning, and Language
EDITED BY William Feindel, M.D.

THIS SYMPOSIUM was arranged with the purpose of cutting across some of the lines dividing various disciplines all having a common interest in different aspects of the functioning of the brain. The essays, given originally as lectures at one of the Jubilee celebrations of the University of Saskatchewan, were deliberately designed to be of interest to laymen concerned with the problem of education as well as to academics dealing daily with products of the brain's activity in teaching and learning. One of the main themes of the book is that the human brain has far greater potentialities than our present methods of education are exploiting; another is that, although our universities can be said to owe their very existence to the multiplex activities of the human mind, the subject of how the brain functions and the application of even our rather meagre knowledge of this field to the sphere of teaching and learning remains greatly neglected in university programmes. The subject of brain function, studied daily by the neurologist and neurosurgeon, should gain the interest of non-medical fields concerned with utilizing the mechanism of the mind.

WILLIAM FEINDEL is William Cone Professor of Neurosurgery, McGill University and the Montreal Neurological Institute, and Attending Neurosurgeon, Royal Victoria Hospital and Catherine Booth Hospital, Montreal. The contributors include members of the faculty of the University of Saskatchewan: PRESIDENT J. W. T. SPINKS; J. F. LEDDY, Dean of Arts and Science; ARTHUR PORTER, Dean of Engineering; and A. HOFFER, Department of Psychiatry. The final essay is contributed by DR. WILDER PENFIELD, Director of the Montreal Neurological institute.

MEMORY,

LEARNING,

and LANGUAGE

The Physical Basis of Mind

Edited by WILLIAM FEINDEL

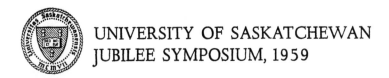

UNIVERSITY OF SASKATCHEWAN
JUBILEE SYMPOSIUM, 1959

UNIVERSITY OF TORONTO PRESS

Copyright, Canada, 1960
University of Toronto Press
London: Oxford University Press
Reprinted 1962, 2017
ISBN 978-1-4875-9850-1 (paper)

FOREWORD

George Bernard Shaw once defined a specialist as one who knows more and more about less and less until eventually he knows everything about nothing. There is, unfortunately, a good deal of truth in this quip. In this symposium, however, we are trying in a modest way to work against this tendency by discussing one subject from the point of view of several disciplines. The theme chosen for the symposium, "Memory, Learning, and Language," is not new; indeed, Dean Leddy, in his historical introduction, gives a broad picture of the evolution of theories of thought during the course of many centuries. Dr. Feindel, in his paper, will then take us into the realm of science as he discusses processes of thought in relation to the structure of the nervous system. Once a relation between thought and the physical structure of the brain is admitted, it is interesting to explore the effect of chemical agents on the brain, and this leads us to Dr. Hoffer's topic, the modification of processes of thought by chemicals. I then do my best to lead our readers up the cybernetic garden path by describing an atomic automaton, but Dr. Porter brings us back to earth by pointing out some of the limitations of so-called thinking machines in his discussion of the mechanical representation of processes of thought. Finally, Dr. Penfield deals with the regions of the human brain concerned with speech.

J. W. T. Spinks

PREFACE

This symposium was arranged as part of a celebration held in September 1959 to mark the fiftieth anniversary of the registration of the first students at the University of Saskatchewan. The speakers—five from the Saskatchewan faculty and one a distinguished guest recognized as a foremost authority on the human brain—represent some of the many academic disciplines which have as a common interest the better understanding of the function of the brain and the application of this understanding to methods of teaching and learning.

Although each of those taking part discusses the physical basis of mind from a specialized point of view, it was intended that the symposium would also be informative and perhaps provocative for a general audience concerned with the broad problems in the field of education.

Presented originally as a verbal symposium, these papers have now been edited and brought together. It is hoped that the publication of this small volume, made possible by a grant provided by the Board of Governors, will help to commemorate the first half-century in the history of the University of Saskatchewan.

During the conversion of this material into a book, any editorial duties on my part were made light by the scholarly help of Dr. J. F. Leddy and by the painstaking and artistic interest shown by the staff of the University of Toronto Press.

WILLIAM FEINDEL

CONTENTS

CONTENTS

Memory, Learning, and Language

AN HISTORICAL INTRODUCTION

by J. F. Leddy

IT SEEMS REASONABLE to suppose that men first became aware of memory as such, differentiating it from other activities of the mind and speculating about its methods of operation, early in human history. Its use is so essential for any connected thought, and any impairment of it through illness, injury, or old age is such an obvious and disturbing phenomenon, that its existence and nature could hardly fail to arouse the curiosity of men with a reflective turn of mind.

Such men were certainly to be found in the early civilizations originating in the river valleys of India and China in the Far East, and of Mesopotamia and Egypt in the Near East, to judge by the already extensive and still increasing literary records found in these areas. However, these records are, in the nature of the case, not sufficiently explicit, so far as our subject is concerned, to delay us until we come to a much later period in the Near East, and not even then in the Far East. Indeed we need not refer again to the latter since the whole current of later Eastern thought, rich and subtle as it proved to be, carried Indian and Chinese speculation away from the individual and the specific, and emphasized the universal and abstract, with consequent indifference to such questions as an analysis of the operations of the human mind.[1]

When the civilizations of the Near East subsided after many centuries, the emergence of the Greeks, in effect the first Europeans, was of dramatic suddenness and brilliance. Within the short space of two centuries, from 550 to 350 B.C.,

[1]F. N. L. Poynter (ed.), *The Brain and Its Functions* (Oxford, 1958), p. 29 ff.

3

the Greeks laid the foundations and erected some of the super-structure of Western thought. In the process they considered and extensively expounded the puzzle of memory, doing so with such effective finality that centuries of effort, up to the beginning of this century, added very little to their basic contribution. Nearly all the basic and general propositions which we have been accustomed to hold with respect to memory were first formulated by or derived from the Greeks and a close examination of many subsequent writers discloses that very often they were simply paraphrasing them. Some of the quotations offered in this paper from various Greek, and Roman, authors establish the modern character of their thought—or rather the traditional character of ours.

Apart from their natural talent for analytic reflection, the Greeks' interest in memory was stimulated by certain charac-teristics of their educational system. The rudimentary schools for the training of scribes in Mesopotamia and Egypt empha-sized constant drill and repetition of the elements. This method was maintained and strengthened in Greek education: "memory work" extended into the later years which were devoted to rhetoric in an effort to train young men to be effective speakers in the courts and public assemblies. Good speakers were assured a place of envied prominence in civic life in Athens and other Greek democracies, and what greater asset could an aspiring orator have than a quick and well-stocked memory? And so there began to appear in Greece in the middle of the fifth century B.C. teachers, many of them itinerant, who professed to have systems to improve the memory. One of them, Hippias, who figures prominently in several of the dialogues of Plato, performed impressive feats of memory himself and undertook to teach others his private system. An interesting summary of such rules, written shortly after 400 B.C., has survived and reminds us of the corres-pondence courses in memory training which are sometimes advertised today. It offers the following rules for memorizing:

First: attend closely
Second: practice
Third: if you hear anything new, associate
          it with what you know[2]

Plato reinforced the Greek inclination to assign a high place to memory in education when he declared many times that a good memory was essential for the philosopher, the man whom he set at the pinnacle of his ideal state. Quite apart from his more technical discussions, to which I shall shortly refer, Plato records in passing a number of shrewd observations on the subject of memory, some possibly original with him, others clearly not so represented. He notes that the memory of children is particularly receptive, saying:

Truly, as is often said, the lessons of our childhood make a wonderful impression on our memories; for I am not sure that I could remember all the discourse of yesterday, but I should be much surprised if I forgot any of these things which I have heard very long ago.[3]

This is a point which much impressed the Greeks and later the Romans, perhaps excessively so, with the result that they established a tradition which generally causes us, even today, to underestimate the capacity of the adult memory. Incidentally, fifteen centuries after Plato, St. Thomas Aquinas, considering this and similar passages in classical literature, offered a charming and unexpected suggestion as to why the memory of children is so effective. We remember best what we find unusual, and for children everything in the world is new and strange.[4]

With a story, allegedly Egyptian, Plato implies that writing is a dubious aid to memory:

At the Egyptian city of Naucratis . . . Theuth . . . was the inventor of many arts . . . but his great discovery was the use of

[2]*Twofold Arguments*, Section 9.
[3]*Timaeus*, 26.
[4]*S.T.*, II–II, 49, 1.

letters. Now in those days . . . Thamus was the King of the whole country of Egypt. . . . To him came Theuth and showed his inventions, desiring that the other Egyptians might be allowed to have the benefit of them. He enumerated them, and Thamus . . . praised some of them and censured others. . . . But when they came to letters, this, said Theuth, will make the Egyptians wiser and give them better memories; it is a specific both for the memory and for the wit. Thamus replied: O most ingenious Theuth, the parent or inventor of an art is not always the best judge of the utility or inutility of his own inventions to the users of them. And in this instance, you who are the father of letters . . . have been led to attribute to them a quality which they cannot have; for this discovery of yours will create forgetfulness in the learners' soul because they will not use their memories; they will trust to the external written characters and not remember of themselves . . . they will be hearers of many things and will have learned nothing; they will be tiresome company, having the show of wisdom without the reality.[5]

One has the uneasy feeling that across the centuries the words of Thamus have some bearing on certain phases of higher education today!

In many matters the Romans were the cultural heirs of the Greeks and in none more so than in the field of rhetoric and education. Cicero, probably the greatest orator in history, wrote a number of treatises on style and rhetoric in which he summarizes the Graeco-Roman tradition in such matters. He gives particular attention to the memory and emphasizes the proposition that a memory can be improved by diligent training and that it will deteriorate if it is not used.[6] Probably the best summary of Greek theories on memory as accepted in Roman educational practice was written at the end of the first century of our era by the schoolmaster Quintilian in his handbook on education. He makes the inevitable point that the memory of children is especially retentive, and maintains that the surest indication of ability in a child is a good

[5]*Phaedrus*, 274–275.
[6]*De Orat.*, 1,5; *Rhet.*, III,16,24.

memory.[7] He concedes, with Cicero, that the memory can be much improved by patient cultivation. He is aware of the vexatious trick of memory in sometimes refusing a recollection when we want it and then casually and suddenly supplying it later when our attention has moved to something else. Like Plato he feels that reliance on written notes can undermine the memory, and he believes it helps the memory if localities or symbols are sharply impressed upon the mind as key associations linked to a particular thought or perception.[8]

None of these observations, of course, leave the realm of accessible generalities at the practical level but they do substantiate the claim that twenty-four centuries ago the Greeks already had as clear a view of the nature and operation of memory as most people acquire today.

However, the Greek philosophers did not stop at this elementary stage but valiantly attempted to answer searching and fundamental questions. How does the memory work, first in storing impressions and secondly in reviving them, as it were, on demand? Why does the memory sometimes make a mistake or fail altogether to respond? What is the difference, if any, between knowledge at its first apprehension and the same knowledge later recalled? In what way does memory differ from imagination in its operation? How is memory related to that elusive faculty, our sense of time?

It would be unfair to Plato and Aristotle to attempt any brief account of their thought on these and similar questions which were expounded in intricate technical detail, but a short reference to one phase of Plato's thought and to another of Aristotle's may be helpful.

Plato offered the following illustration of the way in which memory might work:

[7]Perhaps he makes too much of memory in his appraisal of the young pupil—certainly he would have been scandalized by Nietzsche's maxim that "many a man fails to become a thinker for the sole reason that his memory is too good."
[8]*Orat. Inst.* I,1,19; I,3,1; XI, 2 passim.

I would have you imagine, then, that there exists in the mind of a man a block of wax, which is of different sizes in different men; harder, moister, and having more or less purity in one than another. . . .

Let us say that this tablet is a gift of memory, the mother of the Muses; and that when we wish to remember anything which we have seen, or heard, or thought in our own minds, we hold the wax to the perceptions and thoughts, and in that material receive the impression of them as from the seal of a ring; and that we remember and know what is imprinted as long as the image lasts; but when the image is effaced or cannot be taken, then we forget and do not know.[9]

This analogy of the signet ring on wax was famous and much quoted in ancient times, and may be regarded as the prototype of all subsequent arguments which offer an exclusively mechanical or materialistic explanation for the operation of memory. Plato himself was to find such an approach uncongenial and unsatisfactory and was unable, in the dialogue in which he employed this figure, to reconcile the inherent difficulties in it. None the less, the comparison remained a favourite in the literature of memory for centuries and, of course, has its echoes today in our own general use of the word "impression" in the sense of "notion" or "remembrance."

Aristotle shared Plato's interest in memory and discusses it in several passages in his various works, and also in a short treatise devoted entirely to it. Of a number of interesting points I select one in particular—his attention to the association of ideas, probably the earliest formulation of the subject, if we exclude several hints from Plato. He observes acutely that association proceeds not only by similarity, at which point most of us would terminate the analysis, but also by the contrary and by the contiguous.[10]

Aristotle noted also that memory is a function of "that faculty whereby we perceive time."[11] This theory was especi-

[9]*Theaetetus*, 191 C–D.
[10]*De Memoria et Reminiscentia*, II, cf. Plato, *Phaedo*, 73d–74a.
[11]*De Mem.*, I (at end).

ally agreeable to St. Augustine, the brilliant, powerful, and incisive thinker who lived seven centuries after Aristotle when the Roman power was first crumbling in the West. He gathered up in his own massive scholarship many of the traditions of classical culture and, through his encyclopaedic writings, projected them into the centuries of the Middle Ages, bridging the gap between his own time and the direct rediscovery of the classics during the Renaissance.

Probably the most psychological of the great philosophers, Augustine was deeply preoccupied with the problem of time, perhaps more so than any of his predecessors. He sought to break away from the Greek conception of a remote and ever-lasting cycle, symbolized by the eternal wheeling of the stars in the heavens, and attempted instead to see time as a dimension of the individual soul. Yet time is a most elusive subject for philosophical reflection. As St. Augustine ruefully admits: "What then *is* time? If no one asks me, I know; if I want to explain it to a questioner, I do not know."[12] However, he persevered in his analysis, with some interesting conclusions. For him, all problems of memory were closely entangled with those of time:

The past is memory, the future expectation, the present attention. Or more precisely, since the present is the only one which exists, it follows that the present contains within it the past, as present memory, and the future, as present expectation.[13]

Such an approach to time gives to it a deeply personal and individual significance. Augustine moved to similar conclusions about memory, in particular about what he termed the "inner memory," the place in which knowledge and understanding interact in a special way, the individual becomes most aware of his unique personality, and, in his language, the soul comes to know itself.

[12]*Conf.*, XI, 14.
[13]*Conf.*, XI, 14–20.

Later thinkers have found memory a challenge to understand in terms of their respective systems, especially when they dealt with knowledge. It can be argued that some of them gave answers as significant as those which I have summarized, but for the purposes of this historical and philosophical introduction I am content to suggest that the right questions have been asked for a long time, even if the right answers may still in part elude us.

Theories relating to memory have been remarkably consistent over the centuries with no new major elements until some seventy years ago. In recent decades experimental psychology has enjoyed particular success in elucidating some of the problems of memory or rather of the failure to remember, psychiatry has offered some novel but useful theories, and finally neurology has opened new fields of research. I suspect that in the remainder of this century we may match the initial achievement of the Greeks by eliminating major obscurities which still block our understanding of many aspects of memory. I would judge from recent writers that, *physiologically*, it is likely to remain difficult to account for the persistence of memories[14] and that, *psychologically*, the way in which the memory reconstructs the past continues to be a stubborn problem.[15] Yet we should not be surprised or dismayed to encounter such barriers—in Shakespeare's words, memory is "the warder of the brain."[16] It has so central a place in our thoughts and personalities and is so intimately involved with all our faculties that we cannot expect to unravel its mystery quickly or easily. In its area we are drawing near to the profound issues of life, a fact which ought not to discourage but to stimulate our efforts to know and to understand.

[14]J. S. Wilkie, *The Science of Mind and Brain* (London, 1953), p. 41.
[15]I. M. L. Hunter, *Memory* (London, 1957), p. 152.
[16]*Macbeth* I, 7, 65.

THE BRAIN CONSIDERED AS A THINKING MACHINE

by William Feindel

MAN'S BRAIN will be described in this paper mainly from a structural point of view. This will serve as an anatomical introduction to the following papers which deal with other aspects of the physical basis of the mind.

Dean Leddy's historical review showed that the ancients had profound insight into many of the problems relating to the brain and mind. This is all the more remarkable when we realize that their discussions were based upon a meagre knowledge of the anatomy of the brain. We read, for example, in Aristotle's *De Partibus Animalium* only the safe indication that the "brain in all animals that have one is placed in the front part of the head." Often, too, their anatomical information was erroneous, as when Aristotle described the brain as cold, fluid, and bloodless. We now know that Aristotle's descriptions of brain structure were derived largely from the study of the nervous system in fish and reptiles, but a number of his errors persisted for many centuries. For example, his statement that the brain is the coldest part of the body and "tempers the heat and seething of the heart" was still accepted and taught by the famous William Harvey in the early part of the seventeenth century.

In the second century, following Aristotle, Galen carried out more extensive anatomical studies of the brain but his descriptions also left much to be desired. As a mark of his industry, however, one of the largest veins in the brain is still called after him. It was not until the sixteenth century that the first useful descriptions of the anatomy of the human

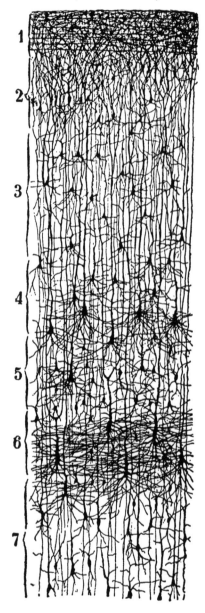

FIGURE 2. Drawing of the numerous nerve cells and fibres (greatly enlarged) in a microscopic sample of grey matter. (From S. Ramon Y Cajal, *Histologie du système nerveux de l'homme et des vertèbres* [Madrid: Consejo Superior De Investigaciones Cientificas, Instituto Ramon Y Cajal, 1955], II, p. 638, Figure 405.)

brain became available from the studies of Leonardo da Vinci, Vesalius, Eustachius, Casserius, and others.

The first serious attempts at correlating the anatomy and pathology of the brain with clinical disorders of brain function, that is, the first proper neurological studies, were made in the later part of the seventeenth century by Thomas Willis and his circle of students and friends at Oxford. As Sherrington says, Thomas Willis "practically refounded the anatomy and physiology of the brain and nerves" and "put the brain and nervous system on a modern footing, so far as that could then be done."[1] In the past fifty years especially, with the aid of the microscope, electronic recording devices, and many ingenious research techniques, great progress has been made in our knowledge of the function of the brain. As in many other scientific fields, the study of the nervous system has never advanced so rapidly as in the past few decades. In spite of this, however, our present understanding of the physical basis of the mind might well be compared to the geographic knowledge of Canada a century and a half before the founding of this university. On a map by Emmanuel Bowen, royal geographer, the western region of Canada could then only be labelled "parts undiscovered." Like the west of that time, man's brain still lies open to further charting by adventurous explorers of the mind.

ANATOMY OF THE BRAIN

This review will be limited to a consideration of three main aspects of the brain: the incredibly complex structure of the human brain; brain electricity or brain waves; and localization of certain specific functions within the brain.

Grey and White Matter

The human brain weighs about three-and-one-half pounds and is about the size of half a loaf of bread. Its surface is a

[1]C. S. S. Sherrington, *Man on his Nature* (Cambridge, 1946), p. 245.

13

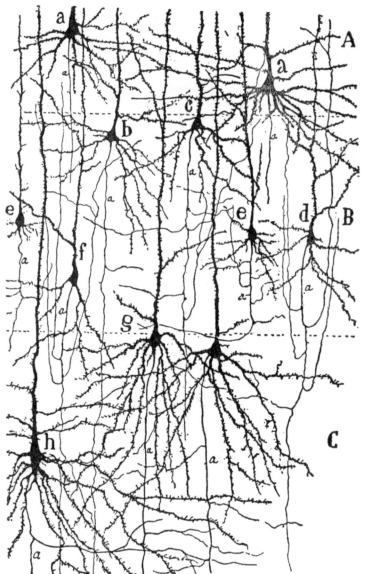

FIGURE 3. Drawing of nerve cells with their numerous processes occurring in the memory cortex of the human brain. (From Cajal, *Histologie du système nerveux de l'homme et des vertèbres,* II, p. 623, Figure 394.)

maze of intricate folds, as though the brain had grown too big for the inside of the skull (Figure 1). These folds, or convolutions, are covered everywhere with a coating of grey matter, the cerebral cortex. The extent of these infoldings is an index of the development of the cerebral cortex in man enormously greater than in any of the subhuman species.

About one-eighth of an inch thick, the cerebral mantle of grey matter consists of millions upon millions of nerve cells (Figure 2). So small that some two hundred of them could be placed across a ten-cent piece, these nerve cells are the microscopic working units of the brain. Each cell has several hundred fine thread-like processes which branch out in a tree-like fashion from a central cell body (Figure 3). These nerve processes, or nerve fibres, fashioned like microscopic conducting wires with an extremely thin insulating layer of fatty material, convey nerve messages throughout the brain. It is these which make up the white matter of the brain substance which lies beneath the cerebral cortex.

What makes the brain so incredibly complex is the fact that it contains more than twelve thousand million nerve cells. These, with their millions and millions of conducting threads, weave a dense feltwork which makes up the substance of the brain. It is indeed a problem to unravel even the simplest pathway in this tangle of connecting nerve threads, which has appropriately been called the "brain jungle."

Thinking Units

The nerve cells are arranged in relays. Each nerve cell has several hundred incoming and several hundred outgoing fibre connections. With a single relay of connections, therefore, one nerve cell may make contact by outgoing messages with some three hundred other cells. These three hundred nerve cells may each in turn make three hundred more connections, to a total of ninety thousand connections, and so on. We know from electrophysiological studies that each relay from one nerve cell to another may occur in one one-thousandth of a second. Theoretically, in four-thousandths of a second, about eight thousand million nerve cells might be engaged from an impulse starting in a single cell. This would represent about three-quarters of the total number of nerve cells in the entire brain. This enormous number of relays may normally never go into action in quite this manner, however, because each cell seems to require far more than one connection to excite it. Nevertheless, this numerical exercise gives a valid idea of the complexity of the network of connections within the brain.

BRAIN WAVES

Every nerve message travelling through the brain seems to be associated with some tiny electrical change. The tiny thinking units, or nerve cells, are in fact like microscopic storage batteries. By magnifying these small electric potentials about a million times by an electronic device, we are able to record them by pens writing on a moving strip of paper or, if we wish, as a sound record on magnetic tape. This is done by placing electric wires on the scalp and leading them through an electronic magnifying device called an electro-encephalograph.

The most prominent type of electrical activity recorded from the brain is rhythmic beating at about ten beats per second. This beating is called alpha activity because it was the first type of brain wave to be successfully recorded. The alpha waves are best seen when the subject is relaxed with his eyes closed and in this sense it is a resting rhythm of the brain. Dean Porter kindly allowed us to record his alpha waves. When his eyes opened, the alpha waves immediately were blocked and replaced by a more rapid type of electrical activity (Figure 4). When the eyes of a subject are closed, the alpha waves may also be arrested if the subject is startled or by mental activity. In the fourth example, the decrease in alpha activity in Dean Porter's record was perhaps due to a

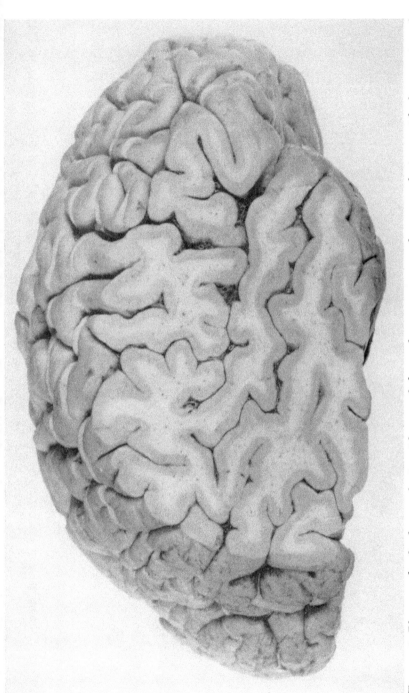

FIGURE 1. Photograph of a human brain with part of the surface cut away to show convolutions, with the covering of grey matter and central core of white matter.

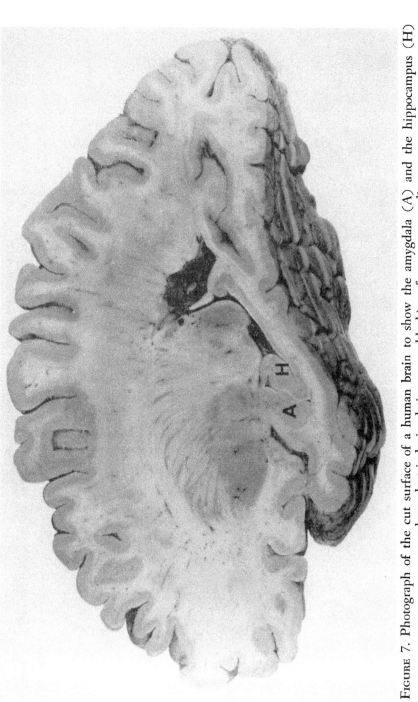

FIGURE 7. Photograph of the cut surface of a human brain to show the amygdala (A) and the hippocampus (H) where electrical stimulation causes blocking of memory recording.

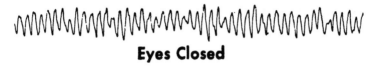

Eyes Closed

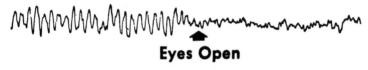

Eyes Open

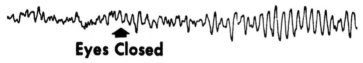

Eyes Closed

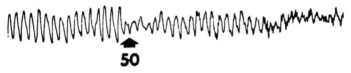

50

FIGURE 4. Records of the electrical activity of the human brain showing (a) normal alpha rhythm, (b) blocking of alpha rhythm by opening the eyes, (c) return of alpha rhythm after closing the eyes, and (d) decrease of alpha rhythm with mental activity.

combination of these two factors, since it occurred just after he was asked what plans he had for the College of Engineering over the next fifty years!

It should be emphasized that this electrical activity seems to be an associated by-product of brain activity and is not necessarily the basis of mental activity or of mind. Its relation to memory, judgment, imagination, and processes of thought is still something of a mystery. At the present time it seems as though the brain waves may tell us no more about the mysteries of the function of the brain than the waves washing on the shore tell us about the mysteries in the depths of the sea.

17

A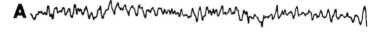

B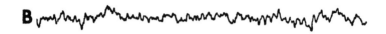

C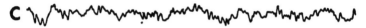

FIGURE 5. Samples of brain electricity recorded from three different subjects as described in the text.

Perhaps another way of illustrating this would be to compare samples of the brain waves from three subjects who, in this case, were a dean of engineering, a professor of neurosurgery, and a baboon. One would note surprisingly little difference in the samples of the three records, allowing for the fact that the baboon was at the disadvantage of being under general anaesthesia (Figure 5). In self-defence, therefore, one would have to conclude that the similarity of these three examples indicates that brain waves are perhaps a rather superficial and even trivial index of the function of the brain! Nevertheless, a vast amount of research activity in the electrical aspects of brain function is going on at the present time and forms a field which I have called before "neuro-engineering." From a practical point of view, the study of brain electricity has led to more critical methods of diagnosis and treatment of certain nervous disorders and has made it possible to map many parts of the human brain.

MAPPING THE BRAIN

In an operation the brain surgeon using a gentle electrical current may stimulate the nerve cells on different parts of the surface of the brain to guide his hand in removing tumors or scars. A by-product of such surgical treatment has been the mapping of the localization of certain specific functions on the cerebral cortex. For example, in the central part of each hemisphere of the brain there is a strip of cortex which is mainly concerned with movements of different parts of the body (Figure 6). Electrical stimulation here may produce discrete movements of individual fingers, or of the arm, face, and so on. The pattern of the parts of the body is arranged in a definite sequence in an upside-down fashion on this motor strip. A similar arrangement can be defined for body sensation on a strip of cortex just behind the motor area. At the back of the brain another cortical area is specialized for visual function and just below the fissure of Sylvius is still another for auditory function.

REMEMBERING AND FORGETTING

Memory is perhaps among the most fascinating subjects now being studied in modern brain research. One should not have to emphasize how basic memory is in relation not only to learning and to language but to education in a very broad sense. It is one of the crucial attributes of mind. Without memory we could not use our brains to store and to recall words and we would, therefore, have no language. If we were unable to remember our experiences—what we see or hear or feel—we would have no learning. It seems obvious then that without language and without learning we would be incapable of thought.

There is another great advantage of memory. As the White Queen said in *Through the Looking Glass*, "It's a poor sort of memory that only works backward." And the White Queen had a point for, with no memory to scan our past experiences, we would be set adrift to live in a meaningless present.

It may be surprising to discover that although memory as a function of the brain has been discussed since ancient times, the particular parts of the human brain concerned with the function of memory have been identified only recently. We have seen that nerve messages shooting through the brain

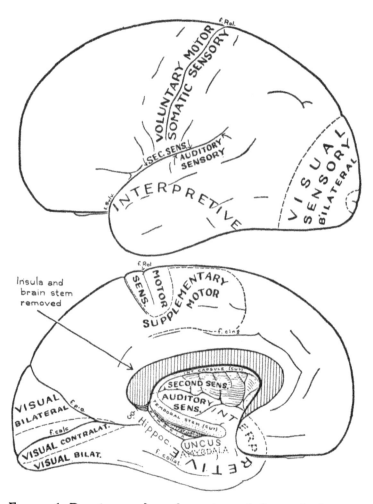

FIGURE 6. Drawing to show the regions of the cerebral cortex concerned with certain specialized functions. (From Wilder Penfield and Lamar Roberts, *Speech and Brain Mechanisms* [Princeton University Press, 1959], p. 41, Figure III–2.)

generate tiny electrical currents. If this process is reversed and an electrical current is applied to the brain, we can artificially excite selected groups of nerve cells concerned with the function of memory, in the same way that responses could be obtained from the motor, sensory, and visual areas of the cerebral cortex.

The two main regions of the brain concerned with memory lie just inside the temple in the portion of the brain called the temporal lobe. If the grey cortex of the brain in this region is stimulated electrically, flashbacks in memory can be produced, as Dr. Penfield has shown, and these memories may in fact be far more vivid than those that can be voluntarily recalled. They are much like the playback from a tape recording, except that they include not only sound but all types of impressions and experiences as well. They seem to be as vivid but not as disorganized as a dream.

In striking contrast to the surface responses, stimulation deeper in the temporal lobe of the brain may suddenly block the experience, subsequently producing a loss of memory for that period of time, or what we call amnesia. The brain structures which seem to be responsible for initiating amnesia have the remarkable names of amygdala and hippocampus— almond and sea-horse—names derived by the early brain anatomists in an imaginative representation of their shape (Figure 7). It has been recognized for many years that certain types of epileptic attacks were associated with amnesia. But it became apparent only recently that these two curious islands of grey matter deep in the temporal lobe were responsible for such memory blocking.

We have mentioned two aspects of memory—recall and recording—but there must also be storage of memory. What is the mechanism? We are still far from a final answer. One explanation is based upon the fact that nerve cells have some of their numerous branches turning back to end on the body of the parent cell, so that they actually receive samplings of their own outgoing messages. For example, see nerve cell *e* in Figure 3. In a sense this is a microscopic feedback or servo-mechanism. It seems quite likely that these self re-exciting nerve loops may keep up a perpetual circular impulse which is the "memory" of that particular cell and continually modifies all messages coming through it in the future. Another explanation relates to the fact that each nerve cell is covered with several hundred tiny button-like endings derived from other nerve cells. Electron microscope studies show that each single button lies intimately against the membrane of the body of the nerve cell. Future research into the physical, chemical, or electrical changes at the site of these tiny buttons will no doubt give us further understanding of the basic processes responsible for the laying down of patterns of memory.

The Brain as a Machine

We hear much today of electronic brains and Dean Porter reviews some of their remarkable accomplishments. In essence, they appear to be electrical systems of memory which at an enormous speed can select specific information in response to the appropriate questions programmed to them by a human operator. But the human brain has certain critical advantages over these electronic devices. It is far more compact. An electronic brain having as many as twelve thousand million thinking units would take up an enormous volume. Even if miniaturized, at the very best an electronic brain would be comparable in size to a very large government grain elevator. The human brain uses a very small amount of electrical energy, something between ten and twenty-five watts. Furthermore, it is portable and comes with a lifetime guarantee!

The word "considered" in the title of this brief review is derived from the Latin "con" meaning together, and "sidera," stars, and means literally "taking the stars together." We hear much today of stars and planets and outer space has captured the imagination of man. But perhaps we would do well to remember that each of us has in his possession the most remarkable of galaxies—twelve billion nerve cells with their myriads of subconstellations in the compact universe of the human brain. It is this inner space of the mind which surely, of all our natural resources, offers the most exciting potentialities. Consideration makes us realize that we are far from exploiting this thinking machine as efficiently as we might in the broad field of creative learning. To paraphrase Cassius, "The fault, dear Brutus, lies not in our brains, but in ourselves, that we are underlings."

MODIFICATION OF PROCESSES OF THOUGHT BY CHEMICALS

by A. Hoffer

CHEMISTS HAVE SELDOM contributed much towards the understanding of thought. That has been the task of philosophers and psychologists. Within our lifetime, however, it has become possible for chemists to influence thought by the development of strange and interesting new chemicals. Yet though it is relatively simple to change processes of thought or thinking by the ingestion of chemicals, it is much more difficult to describe the changes that have occurred. For even though most people know what it means to think, any individual's experience of and with thinking differs to some degree from that of another.

Many philosophers and psychologists have tried to define thought but no definition is generally accepted. Psychiatrists believe that mentally sick people who manifest disorder of thought are more likely than not to suffer from schizophrenia. However, abnormality of thought means many things to many psychiatrists. For the purpose of this discussion I will define thought as the process by which any object (which may be alive, i.e., human, or not alive in a biological sense, i.e., a machine) examines a set of data or information, compares this with other information past or present, and draws a conclusion. This conclusion is judged to be acceptable or not acceptable according to the given values of the object or of society. The decision whether or not to act upon the conclusion so reached is a continuation of the process of thought.

No examples of normal thought are required but perhaps abnormalities of thinking need to be demonstrated. A schizophrenic patient may think he is being watched by the police. This conclusion is based upon the evidence (1) that he saw a patrol car drive by his home, and (2) that he feels people in general are watching him. The patient has disorder of thought because other conclusions are more probable, that is, the patrol car is making a routine run and people do not watch him more than they do other people. His conclusion is wrong but his illness prevents him from judging the adequacy of it.

Such thinking is not creative or productive. Creative thinking allows the individual to see new patterns of relationships in familiar data and to formulate original hypotheses. The creative thinker, as often happens in science, may run into great opposition from other scientists who have not seen the new relationship. But the creative thought must eventually gain support or else the originator has badly misjudged its quality.

Chemicals can alter thought as I have defined it. Since the brain is made up of many chemicals, theoretically any metabolic disorder which disturbs its chemistry may produce disorder of thought. Of particular interest are compounds known as hallucinogens or psychotomimetics, that is, substances which give normal subjects hallucinations and other experiences often undergone by patients who are mentally ill. These chemicals are powerfully active in dosages so small that no toxic changes whatever are induced in the subjects. It is not known whether they induce changes in brain chemistry. They produce changes in perception, in thinking, and in feeling or mood, but do not alter the ability to know where one is, with whom, and at what time. They do not produce unconsciousness or sleep and memory is not impaired. In fact, memory for events long past may be improved. Finally, they are not truth serums.

In general, these chemicals produce two main kinds of experience. The first and best described is the psychotomimetic, which is a laboratory reproduction of many aspects of schizophrenia. The type of disorder of thought present in the man who felt he was being watched by the police is very common and occurs in normal people who are undergoing the psychotomimetic experience. As an experiment I took LSD and had a mild but not unpleasant reaction. My assistants who were watching me wished to give me more LSD but I vigorously refused to take more. After a time I wondered whether I had gone very far into the experience, and if they were extremely concerned about me and wished to give me an antidote, nicotinic acid, to bring me back to reality. They therefore asked me, so I thought, to take more LSD but it was really nicotinic acid I was to get. I was pleased at their concern but they seemed so sad that I was puzzled. An hour later I was given a cup of coffee. It tasted very sour, like nicotinic acid, whereupon I accused them of giving me nicotinic acid in the coffee which they denied. Although I was quite certain that they had given me the antidote, I decided to wait. If I had really taken nicotinic acid I would flush in about an hour. An hour later I did not flush and then realized how abnormal and paranoid my thinking had been.

The psychotomimetic experience may be transient or last throughout most of the day. It is usually very unpleasant and may be frightening. Its only virtue is that it allows us to produce disorders of thought in normal people and the information so derived can be applied to a study of schizophrenia.

The other experience we term psychedelic or mind-manifesting. Thought becomes creative, one's horizons are widened, and the world and its problems are seen with a fresh eye. One of the best of many descriptions, given by Aldous Huxley in *Doors of Perception* relates his experience after receiving 300 mg. of mescaline. We attempt to induce a similar experience in patients who receive these compounds as treatment for disorders of personality. Over half of our patients who achieve a psychedelic experience are subsequently much better people. For example, out of more than half of a series of sixty alcoholics treated in this way over one-half are now sober and good citizens and certainly much happier than they were before. Volunteers who have experienced this type of reaction find to their surprise and pleasure that they are more mature, more tolerant, and have a broader outlook on life. A prominent scientist wrote several months after his experience:

> During the course of reflecting on the experience I've noticed myself "able" to experience intense feelings of love, pride, conceit, shame, hatred, embarrassment, etc.—and I wonder why. These floods of feeling seemed to me to be accompanied by floods of thought and at times they almost seemed to overwhelm me. But this very feeling of being overwhelmed seemed to bring me back to "rationality". These emotional excursions, I think, have given me an "understanding" of myself and other people. They seem to have taught me compassion. I now seem to appreciate Why: why a devout man of the church, a politician, a tyrant, a murderer, an average citizen and why different average citizens.

It is clear then that these chemicals can alter thought as I have defined it, by making one's judgment of conclusions defective or by allowing entirely new and creative conclusions.

The hallucinogenic chemicals include some well known to the public but not to scientists, such as those present in hashish and in the coca plant, and they also include others well known to scientists but not to the public, such as lysergic acid diethylamide (LSD-25) made from rye affected by ergot, or mescaline, the main component of Peyote.

Until recently all the known psychotomimetics were plant chemicals. They resembled adrenaline or adrenaline derivatives. Mescaline is similar to adrenaline. Psilocybin, recently described in *Life*, and ibogaine are indoles, as is adrenolutin which comes from adrenaline. Bulbocapnine is an isoquinoline which is made from adrenaline by some plants. The plant alkaloids may yield either psychotomimetic or psychedelic changes depending upon the psychiatrist and his objectives.

These plant products are, of course, very useful in producing model psychoses and for treatment but are not as interesting as two animal psychotomimetics. These are adrenolutin which I have mentioned as a derivative of adrenaline, and adrenochrome which is chemically between adrenaline and adrenolutin. The animal chemicals produce only psychotomimetic changes but, since these compounds probably are present in the body they are more interesting to students of schizophrenia. We have suggested that an abnormality of adrenochrome metabolism is responsible for the major changes found in schizophrenia.

In the remainder of the paper I will mention some changes in thought produced by LSD, the best known plant hallucinogen, and also by adrenolutin which is similar in activity to adrenochrome. I have already described the type of psychedelic experience produced by LSD and will refer only to the psychotomimetic changes.

In 1953 a volunteer received 100 micrograms of LSD. He had a pleasant and useful experience but as he was returning to reality became quiet and suspicious. At this point, my psychologist and I considered him normal and were making some jest with each other about who would purchase a chocolate bar. This light banter continued for some minutes until the subject in exasperation queried, "Why did you say that?" Later he told us he was convinced that we had played a role for his benefit as a form of test, that we had rehearsed it and acted it for him. Not until the next day would he accept our explanation that it was merely simple chatter.

Almost any change in thought may occur ranging from a complete inability to think because the mind has gone blank to thoughts racing so quickly they outpace the ability to communicate them. Brilliant intellectuals become simple and meek subjects feel that they are omnipotent and can alter the course of humanity itself by a word or deed.

Adrenolutin produces more subtle forms of disorder of thought. Subjects are irritable and impulsive. They quickly jump to conclusions which they proceed to prove by biased observation. One of our volunteers was a very clever graduate doctor. One hour after receiving adrenolutin he was engaged in conversation by a psychiatrist and a psychologist. He was asked his views on state medicine. Immediately he concluded both investigators were Communists. This momentarily surprised him as he had known both of them well and only one looked like a Communist. He still retained some doubt about his conclusion and thereupon determined to test it. He decided to agree with every statement made by either experimenter until he would give them "enough rope to hang themselves." About one hour later the psychologist took up his pencil to make some notes. Upon it was stamped "Government of Saskatchewan." Immediately the subject was sure of his conclusion: who else but a Communist would get a pencil from the Government of Saskatchewan? The next day he was quite disturbed because he was certain he had received an inert substance, that is, a placebo, but if so, how could he account for this type of thinking which he now knew to be abnormal?

I have given a definition of processes of thought, and described briefly some of the well-known chemicals which can modify them. Chemicals are also used to restore normal thought in mentally ill patients but I cannot now enlarge upon this aspect of chemical modification of thought.

The modification of processes of thought by chemicals is a most complicated matter. And thought can create chemicals which modify thought which can produce more chemicals, and so on. The combination of chemistry and psychology which, ten years ago, was considered by many to be a form of insanity, is today considered an important form of creative thinking.

AN ATOMIC AUTOMATON

by J. W. T. Spinks

IN THIS AGE OF AUTOMATION we are all familiar with self-regulating machines, for instance, our houses are kept at constant temperature by using a temperature-regulating device. One of the earliest self-regulating machines to be described (in 1588) was the *baille-blé*, a mechanical device for feeding grain to a flour-mill at a rate depending on the rate of rotation of the millstone which was induced by wind or water.[1] The faster the rate of rotation the faster the grain was fed. This is an example of autoregulation and is at the same time a good example of "feedback," autoregulation being achieved by feedback of information.

Automatic control systems which are actuated by the difference between the actual and desired behaviour of a system and in which some source of external power is introduced, are usually called servomechanisms.[2] The exact definition of a servomechanism is the subject of some dispute: it has been said that it is almost as difficult for the practitioners of servo-techniques to agree on the definition of the servo as it is for a group of theologians to agree on the definition of sin!

In the eighteenth century a number of automats were constructed on completely mechanical lines, and the last thirty years have seen the appearance of a line of synthetic animals which go under the collective name *les petits monstres*.[3] In 1929 a dog, Philidog, was constructed which would follow a path marked out by an electric torch and would turn away

[1]P. Cossa, *La Cybernetique* (Paris: Masson et Cie., 1955).
[2]A. Porter, *An Introduction to Servo-Mechanisms* (London: Methuen, 1950).
[3]Cossa, *La Cybernetique*.

30

and bark if the light came too close. Wiener developed a carriage which was alternately attracted and repelled by light, and in 1948 Grey Walter constructed three famous tortoises, Elsie, Elmer, and Cora, which were also sensitive to light. In 1952 Ducroiq developed two foxes, Job and Barbara, which responded to light and to pressure. Other less playful devices, built for wartime purposes, depended for their action on radar, sound, and heat waves. Obviously, with a little ingenuity, we can build automata which will respond to any desired physical stimuli and a logical development would be to build an atomic automaton.

We have recently built a device called a "crab"[4] which responds to radiation from a radioactive material.[5] Although the crab was built to follow automatically a radioactively tagged soil-burrowing insect (wireworm), the principle evolved would seem to be of rather broader interest. The sensing element in the apparatus is a Geiger tube (Victoreen Co., 1B85) which is rotated about a vertical axis at the end of a fixed arm. The longitudinal axis of the tube lies in a plane parallel to the operating surface (soil). This axis is tangential to the circumference of a circle lying in this plane and about whose centre the arm supporting the Geiger rotates.

If a radioactive source lies on the axis of revolution, the distance between the radioactive source and the Geiger tube will not vary during a revolution, and the counting rate of the Geiger tube per unit angle of revolution will be "constant" except for variations arising from the usual statistical fluctuations associated with radioactive disintegration and background. If, however, the radioactive source does not lie on the axis of revolution, the distance between the tube and the source will vary during a revolution. The count rate generated per unit angle of revolution will not then be "constant"

[4]Pet name, Cy.
[5]B. C. Green and J. W. T. Spinks, *Can. J. Tech.*, **33** (1955), 307–316. See also Scott Russell and L. J. Middleton, *Progress in Nuclear Energy. VI, Biological Sciences* (London): Pergamon Press, 1956), p. 78.

during a revolution, and will tend to be higher in those areas where the Geiger tube is nearer the radioactive source. This variation, which is superimposed on the usual background, can be used to operate a servomechanism, causing the axis of revolution to come closer in line with the radioactive source. The Geiger tube and servomechanism are carried on a free-moving carriage capable of crab-like motion.

All translatory movements of the axis of Geiger revolution are recorded on the operating surface by a stylus which is almost coincident with the axis. A record of the time at which the machine and active source were in a given position is obtained from a clock-driven printing wheel, carrying suitable marking symbols, to represent the time, on its periphery. At chosen intervals this wheel is inked and momentarily pressed against the operating surface. A record of the distance of the radioactive source from the operating surface is also available.

The apparatus described is able to home onto a wireworm, tagged with 20 microcuries of Co^{60}, from a distance of about 15 inches. It is able to follow such a tagged wireworm through 4 inches of soil with an average position error of about one-quarter inch. It is capable of continuous operation at the usual speed for wireworms, a few inches per hour but can, if necessary, travel much faster than this (Figures 1 and 2).

The possibility of using this machine to obtain motion-picture studies of the movements of insects was next investigated.[6] The worm, by means of the tag and the machine, was, in effect, provided with a pencil. The movements of the pencil were photographed using lapse time techniques to give a speeded up picture of the movements of the worm.

A worm was tagged and liberated in a tray of soil placed on the floor. A table was placed over the tray and the machine set on the table. A sheet of glass was placed over the machine. A piece of grease pencil was attached to the machine on the Geiger axis and held in contact with the undersurface of the

[6]B. C. Green and J. W. T. Spinks, *Nature, 181* (1958), 434.

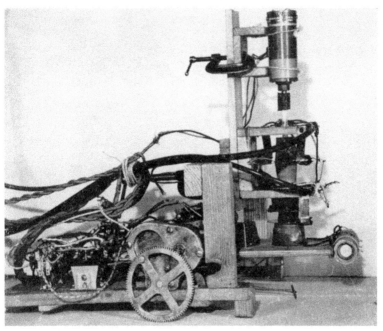

FIGURE 1. Photograph of the early model of the crab.

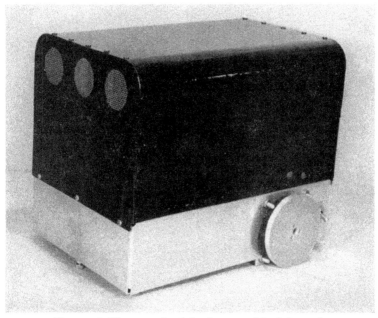

FIGURE 2. Photograph of the later model of the crab.

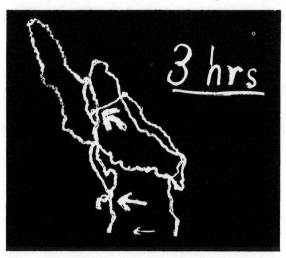

FIGURE 3. Continuous record of the movement of
the wireworm obtained using the crab.

glass by a spring. The path taken by the worm was thus traced
on the lower side of the glass sheet. A 16 mm. motion-picture
camera was mounted above the machine to view it through
the glass sheet. The camera was equipped for solenoid controlled single frame exposures. The solenoid was operated by
a clock-controlled microswitch mounted on the tracking unit.
The exposure interval chosen was 30 seconds and pictures
were taken over a three-hour period. The resulting film gave
what was essentially a speeded up movie of the movements of
the wireworm. As it turned out, the whole operation was
rather abbreviated, and the exposure interval chosen was too
long. However, the short film obtained did demonstrate the
value of the technique. The final picture taken, showing the
path covered in three hours, is shown in Figure 3. The
particular worm involved travelled at the rather high speed of
some 23 inches per hour.

The principle of a rotating Geiger would seem to be capable of numerous other applications, for example, a modifica-

tion of the "crab" has been constructed which will trace out isodose curves.[7]

The foregoing will perhaps have served to introduce you to the latest member of the synthetic family and to the idea that an electronic machine can be constructed capable of exploring, in a limited fashion, the external world.

[7]B. C. Green and J. W. T. Spinks, *Nucleonics*, *16*, No. 4 (1958), 92.

THE MECHANICAL REPRESENTATION OF PROCESSES OF THOUGHT

by *Arthur Porter*

THE IDEA of facilitating human reasoning by mechanical devices is not new. The thirteenth-century Spanish theologian and visionary, Raymond Lull, in his *Ars Magna* described a primitive logic machine and three centuries later the great mathematician, Leibnitz, was of the opinion that the concepts formulated by Lull provided the basis for a universal algebra. Today we can regard the new large-scale calculating machines as direct descendants of Lull's geometrical diagrams and as mechanical representations of the universal algebra to which his ideas gave birth. But the complementary problem of attempting to mechanize even the most elementary processes of thought, although it has attracted widespread attention recently, has not by any means been solved. On the other hand, however, there is a feeling that many of the required components and practical techniques already exist and more profound concepts must be discovered before much progress will be made.

The aim of this paper is to consider briefly the nature of the problem and how far we have advanced in attacking it, and to speculate on the impact of current researches on the evolution of intelligent automata. It is believed that this work is important for two main reasons. First, in many complex processes the optimization of system behaviour inevitably leads to the requirement of self-adapting, or self-organizing, controls and these controls embody essentially a learning capability. Because of these requirements, efforts to imitate mechanically certain characteristics of the nervous system may have an important bearing on the evolution of automation. Secondly, the development of physical models which simulate certain processes of human thought may be useful to medical science. The physical sciences have utilized the model concept so effectively in the past that the method is now regarded as perhaps the most fundamental of research tools and the impact of such concepts in the study of the central nervous system may be appreciable.

It is important to consider initially the nature of processes of thought. For instance, if a process of thought is regarded as being essentially a creative process it can be said, without fear of contradiction, that the mechanization of such a process is not practicable. The question is clearly one of semantics and interpretation. For the purpose of this paper, we will regard processes of thought as involving characteristics such as memory, taking logical decisions, etc. Some of these processes can certainly be mechanized and, indeed, they form the basis of the high-speed calculating machine. However, even though the mechanization of a comparatively lowly form of a process of thought is considered, such as purposeful goal-seeking behaviour, it appears that a machine can handle such problems only after having been programmed by human beings. It is important, therefore, before proceeding further to recognize the limitations of the horizons and to view the problem in the correct perspective. With this end in view it may not be out of place to consider an engineer's idea, expressed in terms of engineering "flow" diagrams of the scheme of dependencies which seem to be involved in processes of thought.

Such a scheme is shown in Figure 1 which, although crude and perhaps even misleading, is intended to distinguish between two major closed cycles of operation. The first is a degenerative cycle involving consciousness, memory, and a process which can be described as conditioning, and the second is a regenerative cycle involving consciousness, memory, learning, thinking, and imagination. The outside stimulant is provided by the environment and clearly there must be cross-coupling between conditioned behaviour and behaviour which involves conscious thought. The degenerative loop portrays habit and it is suggested that too much emphasis on conditioning or drill inevitably leads to a dulling of consciousness; the learning and thinking necessitated in creative pursuits must stimulate consciousness. The importance of this scheme of dependence in considering the mechanization of processes of thought is that, at present, and indeed in the foreseeable future, we can only hope to mechanize the conditioning loop, which is of secondary importance as a process of thought, and there is little possibility that the "creative" loop will be mechanized.

We can extend the relationships indicated in Figure 1 to include external feedback loops which indicate how conditioning and thinking affect the environment—these feedback paths are shown in Figure 2. Again, the minor loop incorporating environment, consciousness, memory, and con-

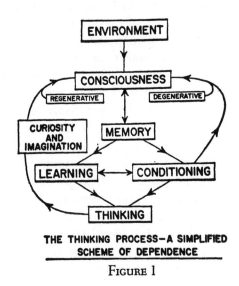

THE THINKING PROCESS—A SIMPLIFIED
SCHEME OF DEPENDENCE

FIGURE 1

37

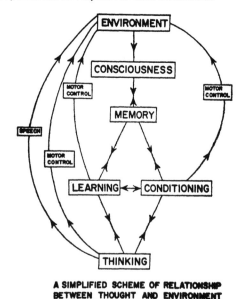

A SIMPLIFIED SCHEME OF RELATIONSHIP
BETWEEN THOUGHT AND ENVIRONMENT

FIGURE 2

ditioning must be regarded as being at a very much lower level of activity of the central nervous system than the loops involving thought. It is perhaps instructive to combine the schemes of dependencies shown in Figures 1 and 2 into a diagram of composite flow as shown in Figure 3. This is highly schematic and is intended to illustrate that processes of thought inevitably must involve appreciably more complexity in the processes of the brain dealing with memory and control than fully or partially conditioned behaviour. In fact, it is convenient to regard the latter as fully programmed controls which suggest inflexibility rather than plasticity. The highly significant role played by "noise generators" in the behaviour of the central and peripheral nervous system is also indicated. More will be said about this subject later.

Even in the most elementary form of thought three basic properties are involved, namely, memory, language, and the

38

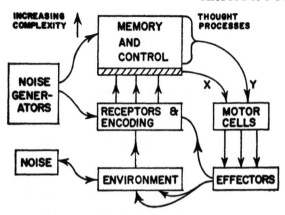

X = FULLY AND PARTIALLY CONDITIONED RESPONSES
(i.e. PROGRAMMED RESPONSES)

Y = HIGH-LEVEL MOTOR RESPONSES
(e.g. SPEECH)

MAJOR FEEDBACK LOOPS IN A
NERVOUS SYSTEM

FIGURE 3

capability of recognizing a pattern. The memory may be of long or short term depending on the nature of the process. The stimulation which excites the process must be converted into a language which can be interpreted by the system, and the system, biological or mechanical, must be endowed with the ability to recognize patterns of language. In processes of thought at a higher level it is probable also that some form of random generator, which initiates inherent "trial and error" procedures, must be involved. There is also the complex phenomenon of "Gestalt." For the present, however, it is convenient to simplify the problem of mechanizing simple processes of thought by considering those in which only memory and language are involved. Such low-level processes of thought may involve: (i) learning of simple motor tasks; (ii) recognition of simple patterns; and (iii) ability to correlate simple processes and to take simple decisions. On the other hand, high-level processes of thought may involve: (i) recognition of spatial and temporal patterns of high complexity; (ii) processes of correlation of a complex kind; (iii) taking complex decisions; and (iv) deductive and inductive reasoning.

A PROGRAMMED PROCESS

A "biological programmed process" may be regarded as one involving the following sequence of events:

environment → consciousness → translation into code → selection of a route → memory →recognition of a pattern → response.

We can simulate some of these transitions in a comparatively simple way. Consider as an example the problem of sorting letters. This does not involve processes of thought at a high level because after the initial period of learning, when the letter sorter has memorized the appropriate postal routing systems, sorting letters becomes essentially a conditioned process. It can be described in terms of a block diagram as shown in Figure 4(i) and the corresponding mechanized process is shown in Figure 4(ii). This is a typical programmed control which embodies the following features.

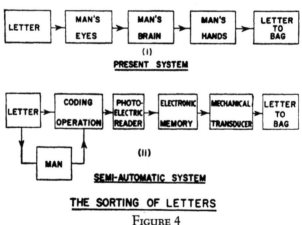

THE SORTING OF LETTERS

FIGURE 4

(i) The only process of thought involved is carried out by a human operator in setting up a code on the letter which describes the address. This is a simple operation but nevertheless one which has not yet been mechanized. The operator is instrumental in causing a sequence of black squares to be printed on the back of the envelope and this is the language which the machine can understand.

(ii) The electronic memory of the machine stores permanently all relevant information concerning the destinations of letters and the corresponding routes, and this information is initially fed into the memory by manual processes. Clearly, the machine must be completely programmed before it will provide meaningful results.

(iii) All the information stored in the memory is scanned continuously and when a pattern of "dots and dashes"[1] appears which corresponds to the identical pattern read on a particular letter the corresponding route code stored in the memory causes, through various electronic and magnetic relays, a gate to open which in turn causes the letter to be deposited in the correct bag. The process of selecting the bag is identical with the process of selecting a line in an automatic telephone exchange.

This simple example demonstrates an important principle in engineering design, that is, to ensure that the man-machine combination is optimum. In this case, the man carries out the elementary coding operation and programmes the memory, and the machine then carries out a purely mechanical task at high speed. In our normal conception of "thought" we would scarcely describe this example as being in the category of mechanized reasoning in spite of the fact that the machine handles a task which, when handled by human operators, involves good memory and exceptional manual dexterity.

The main components in the semi-automatic system of

[1]The "dots" and "dashes" are represented as magnetic patterns on the surface of a magnetic drum.

sorting letters are the magnetic store, consisting perhaps of a magnetic drum upon the surface of which the information concerning destinations and corresponding routes can be "written" in coded form. This information is stored permanently on the drum although if changes are required, due to new postal areas coming into effect for example, these can be readily handled. Although the magnetic storage drum does not by any means operate at high speed as compared, for example, to storage systems using magnetic cores, it is nevertheless an effective method of storage when a large amount of information must be stored and when an access time of the order of one-fiftieth of a second is adequate.

The procedure of coding letters is carried out using a simple keyboard, and each letter of the alphabet has a corresponding code represented by a sequence of dark and blank squares. For example, the letter A is represented by three blank squares followed by one black, the letter B is represented by two blank squares followed by one black and another blank, etc. This simple coding corresponds to the binary numbering system.

The test for coincidence between the input code and the corresponding code written on the drum is obtained by using the principle of conjunction, taking each "digit" at a time. The process of conjunction, which corresponds to the logical connective "and," is very simple to mechanize. Further examples of the mechanization of logical statements will be considered subsequently.

A biological example of a programmed control which bears some resemblance to that above is the mechanism of the "bee's dance." This intricate process does not imply that bees have high intelligence! Indeed the dance can be regarded essentially as a completely programmed operation in which no processes of thought are involved. It should be pointed out that although such programmed processes may not be regarded in them-selves as processes of thought, they are nevertheless prerequisites upon which thought depends and any attempt to mechanize thought will necessarily involve many such programmed processes. The programming may have been learned as a result of a conditioning process or may be inherent in the nervous system.

ARITHMETICAL OPERATIONS

Man's ability to solve complex problems in arithmetic and mathematics is usually regarded as involving thought at a high level. It is in this field that we have had most success in mechanizing processes which frequently tax our brains beyond their limits, not because of the complexity of the task but usually because of the volume of work involved. Nevertheless, the high-speed calculating machines have been devised by human brains and skill and, at the present time, are only capable of carrying out sequences of instructions in accordance with a programme inserted manually.

Mathematics is based on logic and calculating machines are particularly good at simulating logical operations. However, machines carry out arithmetic processes quite differently from a human being. For instance, a human, in performing such processes as addition and multiplication, uses stored multiplication and addition tables which have been implanted in his memory in childhood and which subsequently may be regarded almost as conditioned reflexes. But the machine undertakes arithmetical processes from first principles because it has been found that such methods are appreciably faster than reference to tables; this is a major reason why several recent calculating machines can add two large numbers in a few millionths of a second. The major difference between man and machine in their methods of solving certain types of mathematical problems is that the mathematician, thinking at a high level, frequently discovers short cuts to solutions but the machine must follow slavishly the sequence of operations decided upon by a human programmer.

The problem of language is perhaps the most fundamental of all in considerations relating to the mechanization of processes of thought. Moreover, the process of translating a language into one which a machine can interpret frequently involves very elaborate coding techniques. Perhaps the best example in electronic computer practice at present is introducing into the machine a language designed in such a way that the machine itself virtually carries out its own programming. This is not evidence of intelligent operation, however, because all the steps involved have been anticipated by the design engineer and mathematician in building the machine and in determining its logical operation.

In so far as the process which we can describe as taking logical decisions is concerned we may regard the language of thought as the language of mathematics because both are based on logic. Accordingly, we shall devote some time to the problem of mechanizing the fundamental logical connectives, "and," "or," etc., and of demonstrating how they are used to solve logical goal-seeking problems.

Solving Problems Logically

As an example of a logical problem which has a practical flavour consider the following. A manufacturer can produce a range of twelve products denoted by a, b, c, . . . , k, l. The optimum selections of these products for maximum profit at a particular time will depend upon market conditions which can be defined in terms of logical constraints. If these constraints are as given below, determine the optimum combinations of products:

(i) if a and b and c are selected, or else f or h or j and k together, then d and e together, or g and l together must not be selected.

(ii) i should be selected if a and h and k together or b and f and l together are selected.

Symbolically the problem can be stated as follows:

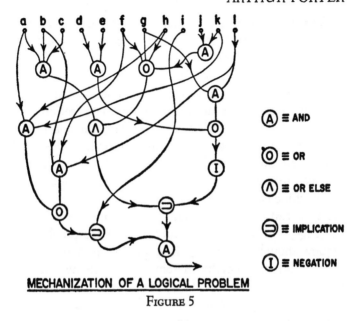

A ≡ AND

O ≡ OR

∧ ≡ OR ELSE

⊖ ≡ IMPLICATION

I ≡ NEGATION

MECHANIZATION OF A LOGICAL PROBLEM

FIGURE 5

(i) $(a.b.c) \wedge (f+h+j.k) \supset (\overline{d.e+g.l})$

(ii) $\quad\quad i \supset (a.h.k+b.f.l)$.

The handling of this problem by pencil and paper methods is very laborious because in effect over four thousand possible combinations must be examined—however, it sometimes is possible to find short cuts. On the other hand, the mechanization of such a problem is quite elementary.[2] We assume that electronic components, usually called decision elements, for simulating the basic logical connectives shown in Figure 5, are available and also that some scanning system capable of scanning automatically through all possible combinations of the variables is available. The interconnection diagram corresponding to this problem is shown in Figure 5, and this is the way in which the demonstration machine has been set up for the solution of this problem.

[2]D. M. McCallum and J. B. Smith, Mechanized Reasoning. *Electronic Engineering* (April, 1951).

Why is a machine so much more effective than man in solving such logical problems? For example, the problem considered above involves five basic steps, namely: (i) Statement of the problem in everyday language. (ii) Translation of (i) above into symbolic language. (iii) Transformation of the symbolic expressions into the appropriate set-up in the machine. (iv) The process of setting-up the machine. (v) The automatic process of obtaining solutions to the problem.

We note that the problem can be mechanized only after it has been formulated by human beings into a language which the machine can handle. But the first four steps above, which must be carried out manually, are required to provide this language, and these are the only steps in the problem which require thought; step (v) is a purely mechanical process which, although lengthy in some cases, can nevertheless be readily programmed. Similarly, the processes involved in programming a digital computer involve steps similar to those given above and here again the important steps are those involving the conversion or translation of language.

Consider another logical problem involving three logical constraints or rules, as given in Figure 6. In the mechanization of such a process we use a set of logical decision elements interconnected as shown in the diagram. But when we know the solution to such a problem we can reduce this comparatively complex array to single logical elements as shown in the diagram. These may correspond to certain classes of neurons although frequently each individual neuron may have as many as five hundred input fibres (i.e., dendrites). Moreover, we know that there is a very large number of such neurons in the human brain and it may be that logical problems are continually being solved by our brains through the mechanism of scanning such neurons until we discover those having an output for a given pattern of input excitation. This is, of course, an extremely crude model of an extremely complex process and it should not be interpreted too literally.

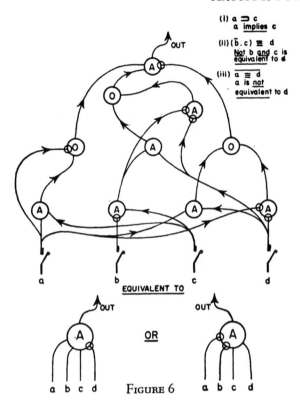

(I) a ⊃ c
  a implies c

(II) (b̄.c) ≡ d
  Not b and c is
  equivalent to d

(iii) a ≢ d
  a is not
  equivalent to d

FIGURE 6

THE MECHANIZATION OF SIMPLE LEARNING PROCEDURES

So far, straightforward programmed processes which have not involved any learning capability on the part of the machine have been considered. Consider now the task of mechanizing processes which cannot be programmed in the normal way. The first step is to examine how a conditioned reflex can be mechanized.

The basic learning process, which characterizes all biological systems and which is probably the essential characteristic for the survival of all biological species, is the process of conditioning.

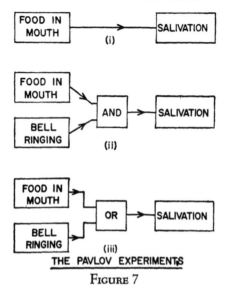

THE PAVLOV EXPERIMENTS

FIGURE 7

The mechanism of animal conditioning is admirably exemplified in the work of Pavlov;[3] a diagrammatic representation of his experiments is given in Figure 7. The main object of the experiments was to show how mental associations between two initially unrelated entities can be formed. For example, a single experience of two contiguous items establishes only a partial connection between them in the nervous system, but additional experiences strengthen the connection until the subject or animal responds to one item upon exposure to the other. Although Pavlov's work brought to light some very complex behaviour on the part of animals, some of which is yet to be explained, from our point of view his conclusions can be summarized as follows: (i) Food in the mouth of a dog is associated with salivation. (ii) If a bell is rung at the same time as food is in the mouth of the dog the result is, naturally, that salivation occurs. If the association between the bell ringing and food in the mouth is repeated a large number of

[3] I. P. Pavlov, *Conditioned Reflexes* (Oxford University Press, 1927).

times, the probability of food in the mouth and the bell ringing is greater than a constant k, and condition (iii), as defined below, applies. (iii) If the bell is rung *or* there is food in the mouth, salivation occurs. It can be concluded that the dog has been conditioned to respond to an external stimulus through a learning process.

Some of the most important work on the mechanization of the process of learning through association has been carried out by Uttley in the development of "self-organizing" automata.[4] Consider the elementary problem of classifying three variables, a, b, and c, which may be regarded as bi-valued states of a system. The "spatial," as opposed to the "temporal," classification of these states can be described in terms of the coincidence units shown schematically in Figure 8. Each coincidence unit incorporates a counter which counts the

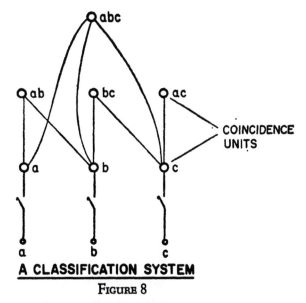

A CLASSIFICATION SYSTEM

FIGURE 8

[4] A. M. Uttley, The Classification of Signals in the Nervous System. *E.E.G. Clin. Neurophysiol.*, *6* (1954), 479.

number of times the unit is excited. A simple extension of the counter provides us with measures of the probabilities, say, of states "a" and "b" occurring simultaneously if "a" alone occurs, etc. In other words the quantity, called the conditional probability of "a" and "b," given a, and similarly the conditional probability of "a" and "b" and "c," etc., can be obtained.

Similarly, if a system can be described by a set of states, a, b, c, d, e, and f, a determination of the frequency with which each state is succeeded by any other state can be used to build up a probability matrix, as shown in Figure 9. After the elapse of sufficient time, and on the assumption that the system is not unduly disturbed by random disturbances, patterns of behaviour will emerge and it will be possible to predict the behaviour of the system on the basis of its

	a	b	c	d	e	f	Next State
a	$\frac{1}{4}$	0	$\frac{1}{4}$	$\frac{1}{2}$	0	0	
b	0	$\frac{1}{2}$	0	0	$\frac{1}{2}$	0	
c	$\frac{1}{3}$	$\frac{1}{6}$	$\frac{1}{6}$	0	$\frac{1}{6}$	$\frac{1}{6}$	
d	$\frac{1}{4}$	0	$\frac{1}{4}$	$\frac{1}{4}$	0	$\frac{1}{4}$	
e	0	0	0	1	0	0	
f	0	$\frac{1}{3}$	$\frac{1}{6}$	0	$\frac{1}{3}$	$\frac{1}{6}$	

Present State

Probability of c following d = $\frac{1}{4}$ etc.

A PROBABILITY MATRIX

FIGURE 9

behaviour in the past; this is a learning process. The transitions from one state to another state can, in fact, be determined on a weighted probability basis.[5]

The above process has been mechanized by Uttley in the form of a so-called conditional probability computer which represents a first step towards the mechanization of learning processes involving many variables, each of which may be many-valued.[6] In contradistinction, the simple process defined by the probability matrix of Figure 9 corresponds essentially to a Markov process, a property of which is that sets of events are connected by a conditional probability that extends over two events only. Obviously, in the nervous system, not only are many events involved in a given process but they will usually have both spatial and temporal patterns associated with them as well.

SELF-ORGANIZING CONTROL SYSTEMS

The study of biological learning systems, coupled with the mechanization of the simple conditioning processes considered previously, will have an important influence on the technology of control systems, especially in connection with the control of complex plants. The key operation at present is the optimization of a process which almost inevitably implies the utilization of data concerning the past behaviour of the process. In order to mechanize optimization we require self-organizing controls which will adapt themselves to their environment. The biological world, in its many manifestations, is made up essentially of such self-adapting systems.

[5]Consider as an elementary example the throwing of a dice, and suppose states a, b, c, . . . , f, correspond to the states of the dice, 1, 2, 3, . . . , 6. If the dice is ideal the probability matrix, after a sufficient number of throws, will consist of elements each of value $1/6$. Alternatively, if the dice is "loaded," or if external influences affect the throwing, the probability matrix may never reach a "steady-state," and a pattern such as that shown in Figure 9 may arise—this particular pattern corresponds, clearly, to an extreme case.

[6]A. M. Uttley, *Conditional Probability Computing in a Nervous System* (N. P. L. Symposium, November 1958; London: Butterworths Press).

Basically, a self-organizing physical controller must operate on the basis of "trial and error," and must store past performance and seek optimum conditions by proceeding always towards the required goal determined by the human operator. Similarly, in biological systems, there is increasing evidence that "random number" generators, which ensure the dynamic behaviour of the self-organizing systems, play as fundamental a part as feedback in biological mechanisms. In addition, therefore, to a conditional probability computer which determines the patterns of behaviour of a system based upon past experience, we have two additional requirements: (i) The system itself must be subjected to random disturbances of an unpredictable nature; otherwise, a self-organizing system would not be necessary. This condition always applies. (ii) Associated with the controlling mechanism must be a "noise generator" which ensures that the principle of "trial and error" is inherent and hence that the system will be goal-directed.

To illustrate the importance of the principle of self-organization in it, consider the evolution of the control of a process. In Figure 10 the three fundamental types of systems of process control are shown diagrammatically. Class (i) exemplifies an ideal process in which it is always possible to predict the behaviour of the process and since no disturbances are involved no feedback is required; in practice, situations such as this never arise. Class (ii) shows the principle of the majority of automatic control systems now in use. To take care of the disturbances inherent in the system a feedback loop is introduced[7] which is completely automatic in operation (cf. a thermostatic control), and in which the human operator decides how the process should be operated by modifying basic control parameters in accordance with his past experience. Class (iii) embodies the normal automatic feedback control which ensures that the "commands" of the computer are carried out and, in addition,

[7]In practice many feedback loops are involved.

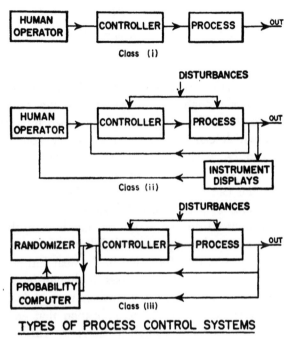

TYPES OF PROCESS CONTROL SYSTEMS

FIGURE 10

a probability computer stores past information and determines the significant conditional probabilities involved in such a process, selects, at random, one or more of the control parameters, changes their values as required by the probability determinations and, in this way, eventually causes the process to operate under optimum conditions.

At present no industrial process is controlled by a truly self-organizing system although it is thought that as research in these fields progresses, the self-organizing principle will be utilized more and more in the future. Perhaps the most important discovery of all from an engineering point of view is that "noise" (i.e., random disturbances) and conditional probability are proving to be the key entities in the control of complex processes.

53

Conclusions

J. Z. Young once stated that "it is convenient to talk about brain function in terms of machine models because we are familiar with machines." An attempt has been made to evaluate progress to date in the mechanization of some elementary processes of thought. It has been shown that only those processes which can be adequately programmed by a human and those which can be described as simple conditioning processes can be mechanized. However, great advances in computer components have been made recently. Electronic storage systems can store hundreds of millions of digits, the switching times of transistorized logical decision elements have been reduced to the order of one-thousandth of a millionth of a second, component reliability is increasing, and it is not improbable, therefore, that in the near future means will be found to mechanize processes of thought at a somewhat higher level than those with which we are dealing at present. Nevertheless, there is no indication that creativity, the most important manifestation of thought, will be mechanized for a long time to come.

Present research in the field of mechanizing processes of thought is already having an important impact on the control of complex industrial and commercial processes and it exemplifies very strongly the importance of encouraging interdisciplinary research of this kind.

THE NATURE OF SPEECH

by Wilder Penfield

THE MEMBERS OF THIS SYMPOSIUM have been discussing *the physical basis of the mind* with special emphasis on memory, learning, and language. It is hard to imagine a more appropriate topic for the Golden Jubilee of the University of Saskatchewan, although we are not likely to answer all the questions raised, not today, nor tomorrow, nor even in a thousand years.

Dean Leddy, with keen insight into their thinking on this subject, helped us to look back at the Greeks of twenty-four centuries ago. We have advanced a little since then; but surprisingly little. Socrates, had he been at the Jubilee, could have argued some points to good purpose. He might have asked questions that would have made us blush.

Four hundred and fifty years from now, when the University of Saskatchewan comes to its five hundredth convocation, I suppose some unsettled problems will concern the faculty still. Perhaps then a future president will declare a second Golden Jubilee and bid a future dean discuss again the human brain and its relation to the mind of man—and to God.

Perhaps, in that happy far off day, Communism and Capitalism will have been put to bed together, giving issue to better ways of life in a sane new world. But whatever changes come to ideologies and creeds and governments, I predict that universities will survive and grow in depth and height and influence. Since they first raised their heads through the haze of the mediaeval renaissance, they have altered little. Eight centuries have passed over them in their steady growth, while churches changed and rulers rose and fell. Universities hold to one steadying purpose through the years: to seek the truth and to teach it.

Men talk of madness in the world in which we live, and of the destruction that threatens us now. They forget that truth has power to set us free, power to show the way to peace and to lead man into a sane new world. Let them, then, bid their governments give the universities full support, and with it freedom, financial independence. Then universities will bring forth from science good, not evil, and from the humanities, understanding. Our task meanwhile is to learn to understand the mind of man before it is too late.

When the five hundredth convocation does come to Saskatoon, in the year of our Lord 2409, physiologists will at least know more about the patterns of the pathways in the brain, patterns through which electrical potentials must flash to make the background of a thought. But I suspect that they will wonder still, as we do now, how it is that nerve impulse becomes a thought and thought, in turn, electrical potential. They will wonder still what lies beyond the grave, and strive to read the will of God in the planning of the basis of the mind.

Functional Anatomy

My task in this symposium is to consider the nature of speech. Speech, above all else, separates us from the other animals, and lifts us above them. It seems reasonable to conclude then that there must be in the human brain some special mechanism that makes speech possible, a mechanism which not even our friend the dog shares with us, nor the anthropoid ape.

Professor Feindel discussed the structure of the human nervous system, describing functional units within the brain and indicating which areas of the cerebral cortex are chiefly devoted to the separate forms of sensation and which to the voluntary control of movement. All these areas may be

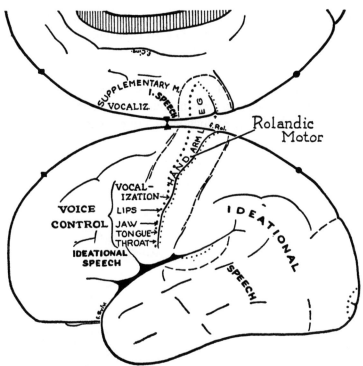

FIGURE 1. Diagram of left hemisphere of cerebral cortex of man. Motor areas devoted to voluntary voice control are indicated and would be the same in homologous areas of the other hemisphere. Vocalization can also be produced by stimulation in the supplementary motor area of both hemispheres.

The areas devoted to ideational elaboration of speech which are quite separate from the above are normally found only in the left hemisphere. (From W. Penfield and L. Roberts, *Speech and Brain-Mechanisms* [Princeton University Press, 1959].)

identified in other mammals, with certain exceptions, by one technique or another.

In man vocalization can be produced by gentle electrical stimulation in motor and supplementary motor areas of the cerebral cortex, as shown in Figure 1. Stimulation of these cortical areas does not produce vocalization in laboratory mammals. The dog and the cow and the monkey each uses his voice to suit his particular purpose, but does so through other pathways in the brain which need not concern us now.

Aside from motor control, for the ideational requirements of speech man uses certain areas in the cortex of one hemisphere, normally in the left one which is therefore called the dominant

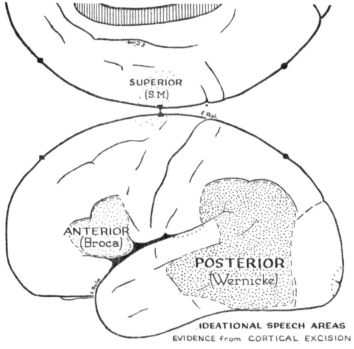

FIGURE 2. Areas devoted to ideational elaboration of speech in the left hemisphere. Aphasia follows injury to any of these areas. It is of short duration when the superior area alone is involved; much longer when the anterior area is injured, and it may be permanent if the posterior area is destroyed, except in the case of children. A child in the first ten years of life, after severe brain injury, may transfer speech function to the opposite hemisphere with a perfect result. (Penfield and Roberts, 1959.)

hemisphere. These ideational areas are employed when he speaks or writes, and when he reads or listens to the speech of others.

The posterior speech area originally discovered by Wernicke (1874) is the most important (Figure 2). The anterior speech area discovered by Broca in 1861 is also important but seems to be less indispensable. The superior speech area is least important. All three are joined together into a functional unit by their projection connections to the thalamus of the same side (Figure 3).

I propose to discuss speech from a psychological point of view after the briefest review of experience in electrical stimulation of the cerebral cortex of conscious men. The procedures

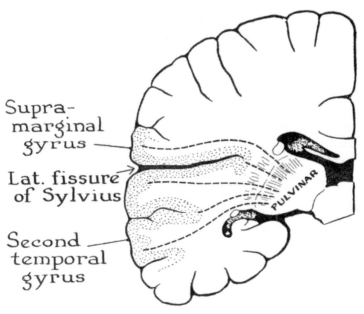

SUBCORTICAL PROJECTION
to SPEECH CORTEX

FIGURE 3. Diagram of connections of posterior speech cortex with underlying thalamus (pulvinar). (Penfield and Roberts, 1959.)

are not experiments and are not painful. They serve a useful purpose before surgical treatment is carried out. Some areas respond positively to the application of an electrode carrying a gentle electrical current. Others do not.

Stimulation of the motor convolution (Figure 4) may cause the opposite hand to move or the voice to be employed in a vowel sound. Stimulation of a sensory area of the cortex may cause the patient to see lights, hear elementary sounds, feel tingling or movement in some part of the body. Stimulation of the interpretive cortex on the temporal lobe of either side may cause the patient to re-experience those things to which he paid attention in some previous period of time, hearing and seeing the things he then heard and saw.

But when an electrode is applied to one of the three cortical speech areas, neither words nor thoughts of words are produced. The current is apt to interfere with the speech mechanism. The patient is not aware of this unless he needs to use the mechanism. Then he discovers to his surprise that he cannot speak or that he can use some words but seems to have lost others, especially the names of things. The same is true when one of these areas is injured or pressed upon. This disturbance is called aphasia, or dysphasia. During it there is difficulty in speaking, writing, or understanding words. Aphasia may be defined briefly as a difficulty in the ideational elaboration of speech and in the comprehension of the meaning of words previously familiar. When interference is not complete there is usually misuse of words, or the patient employs circuitous substitution of words. Most characteristic of all, there is apt to be perseveration. That is, the subject continues to employ a word which does not suit the meaning intended, although it may have been appropriate the first time it was used.

If a gentle electrical current is applied to any one of the three speech areas of the exposed cerebral cortex, the patient may lose capacity to speak, to a greater or lesser extent. He is

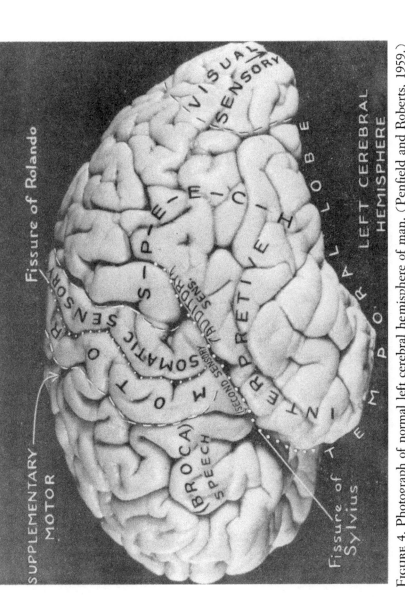

FIGURE 4. Photograph of normal left cerebral hemisphere of man. (Penfield and Roberts, 1959.)

aphasic. But he only discovers this when he tries to speak or perhaps to understand speech. Other mechanisms of the brain are apparently not affected. Dr. Lamar Roberts and I have made practical use of this, in hundreds of cases, to map out areas devoted to speech.

PSYCHOLOGY

The intelligent patients who lie on the operating table, unable to see the operative field, but keenly introspective, can teach us something. We have recorded their words carefully through the years. Let me refer to the case of C. H., which we have described in an earlier publication, and proceed from that to a discussion of mechanisms.

Case C. H.

After the injection of local anaesthetic, the left hemisphere was exposed (Figure 5) preparatory to the removal of a temporal lobe scar. We set out to map the speech areas so as to avoid injuring them. The patient, whose face and eyes were shielded by a little tent, was shown small pictures, one after another. He named each in turn. He had no means of knowing when the surgeon's electrode was applied to the brain or when it was removed.

The electrode was applied to the cortex at the point where ticket 26 was dropped. This was on the anterior speech area. Meanwhile he was being shown a picture of a human foot. "Oh," he said, "I know what that is." After a pause, he added: "That is what you put in your shoes." The electrode was then withdrawn and he exclaimed suddenly, "Foot." The speech mechanism had only been partly put out of use. He could not recall the word "foot," so had used a circumlocution to present his meaning.

The electrode was applied at 28, in the posterior speech area, and simultaneously he was shown a picture of a butterfly. In this case the electric current seemed to block the speech mechanism almost completely and he was silent. He remained

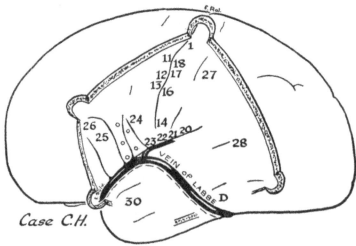

FIGURE 5. Case C. H. Drawing of field of operation within the craniotomy opening. The numbers indicate points at which electrical stimulation produced a demonstrable effect. Numbers 11, 12, and 13 are on the precentral motor gyrus and 1, 18, 17, 16, and 14 are on the sensory postcentral gyrus. At 12 and 13 stimulation produced movement of the jaw; at 24 movement of the mouth. At 26, 27, and 28 the electric current produced aphasia.

so, although Dr. Pasquet, who was showing the pictures, pressed for an answer and asked why he did not reply. He did shake his head and say, "No." As the electrode was withdrawn, there was after-discharge, as shown by recording electrodes. He was completely silent then. The after-discharge disappeared suddenly and he spoke at once: "Now I can talk —butterfly. I couldn't get that word, butterfly, and then I tried to get the word, moth." In this case the speech mechanism was so nearly completely blocked at first that he could only say "No." Then the block became complete and he was silent. But he was able to snap his fingers in exasperation, though he could not speak and probably could not have used his fingers to write, had he had a pencil.

It is obvious that he understood what he saw while aphasic. He must have presented the concept "butterfly" to the speech mechanism but the word did not come. So he substituted the idea of a moth but "drew a blank" once more. It is clear that C. H. retained control of some mechanism by which he could compare the concept of a butterfly to that of a moth and could appreciate the resemblance between them. This suggests that, under normal circumstances, in the process of naming, a man must present to the speech mechanism a concept, or a proposition, and some automatic type of reflex produces for him the correct name instantly. One must conclude, then, that there is another mechanism within the brain that is independent of speech, a *concept mechanism*. C. H. saw a particular butterfly and summoned the corresponding general concept. When this elicited nothing but silence from the speech mechanism, he passed on to moth and was again disappointed.

Instead of a butterfly, he might have seen at that time the face of a friend peering at him under his little tent. If so, he would have summoned the generalized concept of that friend derived from previous meetings. He would have presented the concept to his speech mechanism in the expectation that the proper name, John Jones for example, would be forthcoming. He would have been disappointed by his aphasia.

This, then, should throw some light on the ideational process that is prerequisite to normal speaking. It is clear that at least two physiological mechanisms or processes are involved: first, the recognition of a "remembered" concept and second, the production of a "remembered" word.

Hughlings Jackson coined the expression "verbalizing." Speech, he said, was the second half of the dual process of verbalizing. The first half was perception. Speaking, therefore, would require perception followed by verbalizing. The comprehension of what others might say would, I suppose, be called de-verbalizing.

It is clear that C. H. was able to perceive, that is, to see the picture and pass from it to the general concept of butterfly. When the word did not come automatically he was able to try the voluntary act of substitution. At least, he would consider the substitution a voluntary act, not a reflex, if he had been asked. And he was able to carry out the voluntary movement of snapping his fingers to convey his meaning when words failed him. For that purpose, apparently, he did not need to call on the speech mechanism.

This argues for the existence within the brain of a central co-ordinating or integrating system, through which a person is able to transform sense impression into concept. That is the process of perception. C. H. was able to turn back and forth from concept mechanism to speech mechanism, thanks to those centrencephalic integrating circuits which obviously operate back and forth through brainstem and cortex. These alone could make such co-ordinated activity possible.

MEMORY MECHANISMS

Memory is a term used loosely to include more than one process. Various brain mechanisms are involved in it: first, the memory of individual experiences;[1] second, memory of concepts or generalizations; and third, memory of words. It is obvious that as the years pass a ganglionic record is formed for each type of possible recall. The evidence from electrical stimulation of the cortex in conscious man makes it clear that these records depend on functionally separable neurone mechanics.

LEARNING TO SPEAK

Consider the beginning of learning a language. In the second year of life the child is taught the mother tongue by the direct method, the mother's method. According to Leopold, there is, at this stage, a lag of about two to seven

[1]For a discussion of experiential recall see W. Penfield, The interpretive cortex. *Science*, *129* (June 26, 1959), pp. 1719–25.

months from the first hearing of a word until the child's first meaningful utterance.[2] In that interval the child must establish a concept of the thing to be named. He must also create a neurone counterpart of the name in which is included both the sound and the motor pattern that will produce the name or something like it. The pattern of a word, both motor and sensory, must be established somehow in the speech mechanism of the dominant hemisphere. The concept must also be set up somewhere in the neurone system which, as we have seen, is functionally separable from speech. We have at present no knowledge of where the neurone circuits of that concept system or mechanism are located.

Take a simple example which I have used before:[3] Each time a mother prepares to take her child out of doors she may say "go bye-bye" (a word in the specialized vocabulary of baby-talk with the authority of the mothers of the race behind it). Before the child can begin to name that proposition for himself, he must learn to understand the meaning of the concept of going out of doors. He must make a generalization from a number of particular experiences in which he was taken out of doors in his baby carriage. One may surmise that this concept is eventually recorded in a patterned unit. The pattern is produced by the passage of a sequence of electrical potentials through nerve cells and their connections to other neurones within the speech areas of the brain. Each passage of the stream of impulses in that pattern must leave behind some persisting facilitation which will in time form a sort of habit unit. This, it may be assumed, is the physical basis of the concept of going out of doors, the basis of one type of memory, the memory of concepts.

The time comes when the child has established the concept of going out of doors and he recognizes the sound of the

[2]W. Leopold, *Speech Development of a Bilingual Child* (Evanston, Ill.: Northwestern University Press, 1939).

[3]W. Penfield and L. Roberts, *Speech and Brain-Mechanisms* (Princeton University Press, 1959).

phrase "go bye-bye." When the mother speaks the words he laughs, showing his pleasure at the prospect. An intelligent dog might well be equal to the child at this point and might wag his tail at the sound of the words. Pavlov, the great Russian physiologist, would say that the dog has formed a "conditioned reflex." All learning may well be based on the establishment of what he called a conditioned reflex, in some form and some place within the brain.

But the child comes to the time when he will take a remarkable step. It is, in a way, the human miracle. No dog or parrot can follow him here, for he will speak the words, "go bye-bye," and know what they mean. His mother, no doubt, will cry out in admiration, as she should, though no one else would probably have recognized the lisping sounds. The child has presented a concept to his speech mechanism which, in turn, presented him with awareness of what the sound would be like. To the sound the child now adds the way of imitation. The sound pattern and the motor verbal pattern are forming in the area of the brain which man devotes to speech. The unit is not final yet, for the speech mechanism is plastic and will remain so for some years. He will modify his record of the sound and improve the pattern of his pronunciation. He will modify the record of the concept too, as baby carriage is replaced by other means of locomotion.

Let us reconsider the concept, "butterfly," and how it formed itself in the mind of the adult, C. H. He first saw this creature, no doubt, as a child when he ran through some meadow. The lovely coloured fluttering thing passed him by and his mother said, "It's a butterfly." Another day he may have seen one light on a flower nearby and may have locked at its wings and seen how they went, while someone watching said the word, "butterfly, butterfly." And he smiled and said the word himself. Then, later on, he discovered another one in a picture at kindergarten and knew it for a butterfly. In adult life he had forgotten the individual butterflies he had seen. The record of each adventure with this fluttering object had faded far beyond the limits of voluntary recall. But the generalization, the concept of a butterfly, remained. This concept is what we would call a memory, of course, but it is quite different from the memory one has of individual experiences, different in the sense that it is a generalization. Individual experiences are kept in an experiential record of the particular time sequences. This record is forever fading from conscious memory unless some emotion or meaning makes a particular strip of time memorable. The record of generalizations of concepts, drawn from the stream of successive experience does not fade, but goes with us through life. And this, no doubt, keeps us from the confusion of remembering too much.

When C. H., under normal circumstances, conjured up within himself the concept "butterfly," the word came to him at once and he could speak it. When he heard the word, the concept flashed into his consciousness. There was an instantaneous automatic reflex between the word unit and the concept unit. It operated in either direction. The concept was summoned with equal facility when he heard the word or read it. In time, he could seem to ignore everything but the concept. If he were bilingual he might not be aware in what language he had read or heard the word. He could focus attention on meaning and no longer be aware of the reflex actions that were now serving him so well, until the speech mechanism was suddenly blocked. Then he was left with perception and concept only; aphasia blocked his access to the word.

Speaking is not just the simple reverse of listening to talk or reading it. When an adult summons the idea of a butterfly and names it, the automatic reflex activation passes from the concept unit within the brain to a verbal unit pattern within the speech mechanism. That pattern makes the Canadian speak the word, as he has heard it, and the Englishman as he has heard it. They pronounce butterfly quite differently.

There is then, within the speech mechanism of the dominant hemisphere, a sound pattern and a speaking or verbal pattern. They are closely related, but very different in structure. When the child reaches the later years of the first decade of life, he comes to the period of expansion of vocabulary. He then adds words, and concepts too, with amazing rapidity. He seems to borrow basic sound units and verbal units from the words already learned in the language. If he heard English and French, and Russian too, early enough, he could expand in each language separately, with equal ease and perfect accent. He could do this because he had developed a set of units and a general framework for each language while the speech mechanism was still plastic. Neither Chinese pronunciation, nor any other, holds terrors for an Anglo-Saxon child when he is young enough and his speech brain is still plastic.

Naming, then, requires recognition of concepts and reflex linkage with the related words. At the outset, speech is only naming. Later, it is more than that. But this lightning swift reflex linkage, that works in either direction between concept and word, word and concept, remains the essential element in speaking, writing, reading, and understanding speech.

In later decades of life the physiology of language learning is altered. To meet the new problem, teachers commonly employ an indirect technique of instruction, quite different from the mother's method. Present-day education in the secondary living languages has been patterned on the methods devised to teach the dead languages. The result falls far short of what might be achieved if educators would give due consideration to the physical basis of the mind. There is a biological time-table in the evolution of each human brain that might teach the teacher when to teach and how.

In conclusion, it is clear that there are numerous neurone

mechanisms within the brain which are specialized to various uses. Some of them, at least, are functionally separable and all of them are probably controlled in varying combinations through a central integrating and co-ordinating system.

We have not had the opportunity to go deeply into all the problems this topic suggests. But, at least, we have looked at the place in the brain from which words come, and drawn some meaning from new evidence that has to do with the nature of speech. And ability to speak is the gift that has lifted man above the other mammals.

9 781487 598501